# FREEDOM
# FROM FAT

# FREEDOM FROM FAT

FIGHT BIG GOVERNMENT AND BIG FOOD'S
CONSPIRACY TO KEEP YOU OVERWEIGHT —
FLIP ON YOUR NATURAL FAT-BURNING SWITCH

**BRAD LEMLEY**

# TABLE OF CONTENTS

# INTRODUCTION:
## Revelation, Courtesy of Three Young Clerks

Last week, at my local big-box hardware store—of all places—I had a soul-shaking epiphany.

I couldn't find the paint I wanted, so a friendly young clerk directed me to the right aisle.

Then, in the garden department, a helpful employee gave me advice on shade-tolerant plants.

Finally, a young woman efficiently rang up my humble collection of weekend-warrior accouterments.

Mundane stuff, right? But here's the thing. Each of these people was under 30 years old.

*And each of them weighed well over 250 pounds!*

Actually, the two guys were easily north of 300. The girl was the slimmest of the bunch, at—I'd estimate—5-foot-2 and 275 pounds.

Now . . . I almost didn't process this as unusual. Every day in America, morbidly obese people are everywhere.

But on this particular afternoon, I was struck by an amazing, undeniable revelation. The fact that I'd met three dangerously overweight young adults in quick succession underscored the fact that obesity is absolutely epidemic.

If these three young people had been born in any time period except the last three decades, and in any country but America, their chances of becoming so massively fat would have been extremely—so to speak—slim.

But this trio had the great misfortune of being born in the middle of a perverted food culture, one in which the worst foods are cheap and ubiquitous and the best ones expensive and scarce.

Worse, they all had no doubt suffered from a lifetime of precisely backward weight-loss "advice." My guess is that they had dutifully avoided eating fat (especially butter!), consumed lots of diet soda and "heart-healthy" whole grains, and all the while wondered despairingly as they got thicker and rounder for their pains.

The more I thought about it, the angrier I got.

At this rate, these people were likely to die young from Type 2 diabetes—an exceptionally awful way to go, as it is typically preceded by blindness, amputation, and other horrors. They were part of a blighted generation, destined—for the first time in American history—to have shorter life spans than their parents.

So . . . here we are, my friend.

Perhaps the culture has done a number on your and your family as well, leaving you and your loved ones ever heavier despite vigorous efforts to follow the mainstream's advice.

If so, the solution is simple.

Forget what you've been told and pay attention to the information in this exclusive collection of "Freedom From Fat" guides.

The advice you'll find here is firmly rooted in real, cutting-edge science, not profit-driven Big Food and Big Government spin.

You'll discover:

- Why counting calories does not work, but counting *this* does
- Which foods boost your fat-burning potential
- The one dietary change you must make to start dropping pounds
- An exercise secret that will turbocharge your fat loss.

Don't be a victim. A slim, healthy, vibrant body can be yours, but you need to think your way there.

These guides will show you the way.

Enjoy the journey. I wish you every success. And if I can think of a diplomatic way to do it, I'll slip copies of these guides to the nice young people at my hardware store.

Best,

Brad Lemley

# SIN FOODS FOR HEALTHY LIVING

What are the basic rules of healthy eating?

Most people would be quick to answer that question with the most popular answers. Stick to low-fat products. Avoid red meat at all costs, and choose chicken or fish instead. Keep an eye on your cholesterol. Above all else, keep the butter off the table.

This is what I used to think as well. How could I not, when these solutions are touted everywhere?

I've written this report to show you that a great deal of what we've been taught about nutrition for the last 40 years has been wrong.

After nearly 30 years of working as a health and science writer, it's clear to me that most of the advice doled out by the American Heart Association, the National Institutes of Health, and the U.S. Department of Agriculture has been inherently misleading.

This problem didn't spring up overnight. It's slowly overtaken medicine, politics, and popular opinion for two generations.

In the 1950s and '60s, the country was in a panic about how to tackle the growing rate of heart disease. In the scramble that ensued, leading scientists and nutritionists tried to provide an explanation. They decreed that we needed to cut out saturated fat and cholesterol, ideas that have permeated our culture ever since.

The problem was, the "evidence" that backed up these claims was a chaotic mess of assumptions and poorly executed studies, all based more on food industry political influence than scientific fact.

How do we know this? Just look at the results! After more than half a century of recommending a low-fat, high-carbohydrate diet to the American public, our health has gone from bad to much, much worse.

Heart disease is now the leading cause of death for both men and women. Obesity has become an epidemic, affecting one in three American adults—it was only one in seven in 1961. Diabetes has skyrocketed, from less than 1% of adults to more than 11% today.

These health issues are a direct result of our diets.

So many of us struggle with our weight and our health. Years of diets and exercise never seem to help melt the pounds away. We fight through breakfasts of cottage cheese and fruit, trade our steak and potatoes for salads and rice, and somehow get fatter, sicker, and sadder.

What if I told you that none of that is your fault? That your diet isn't working because you've been misled about what your body needs to be strong, slender, and healthy?

Contrary to what we have been told, we should be eating more protein and animal fat and less grains and carbohydrates. Milk, eggs, meat, and cheese are far better for you than pasta, bread, cereal, and other grains. And a diet based in fruits and vegetables simply cannot make up for healthy animal fats. In fact, recent studies have shown that any kind of carbohydrates are unhealthy. That includes whole grains, as well as starchy vegetables and fruits.

The war that the National Institutes of Health launched against saturated fats was rooted in unproven theories and skewed data. It led to harmful substances like liquid seed oils (corn, soy, canola) and artificially hardened "trans" fats in our diets. Although the dangers of those are becoming better known, many of the nutritional "facts" still being taught are detrimental to our health and development.

Unfortunately, the media still support the nutrition mainstream and harp on the same old points that have now been disproven.

My goal is simple: to help you to realize that you no longer have to avoid the foods that you love. Don't shy away from red meat. Cover your vegetables in butter. Leave the fruit and fat-free yogurt behind and dive into a plate of bacon and eggs for breakfast.

Trust me—you'll thank me in the long run.

Here's my list of "sin foods" that not only taste good, but are good for your health. I hope that it leads you to robust health and happiness, just as it has for me!

## LEARNING FROM HISTORY

Think of human history as a 100-yard football field. In the documentary *The Perfect Human Diet*, American scientist Dr. Loren Cordain explains that the first humans anatomically similar to us, known as homo erectus, appeared 2 million years ago at the zero yard line.

Humans walked 99½ yards of that football field eating a high protein and animal diet. Agriculture began only 10,000 years ago. This means grains, legumes, and dairy products were introduced in a major way to our diets only on the half-yard line!

And today? Sugars, wheat, and vegetable oil extracted from seeds such as soybeans and corn make up 70% of the calories we eat. These processed foods didn't become part of our diet until the 1900s, which puts them at the 0.001-yard line!

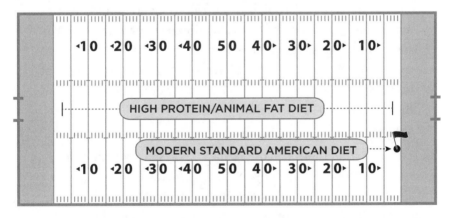

Since that time, life spans have lengthened due to the conquest of infectious disease, but our years of active, robust, productive health have done nothing but decline. As we continue to ignore the diets that kept us thriving and evolving throughout human history, the results become more severe.

The fact is now clearly established that the low-fat, high-carb diet is a nutritional nightmare. Just look at the soaring obesity and diabetes rates since 1980, when the federal government first began actively promoting this way of eating.

But if it's so wrong, why has it hung on? In a word, money. There is much more profit to be made by selling 4 cents worth of commodity wheat in a $4 box of Wheaties than there is in selling fresh meats and vegetables.

Grains—especially when propped up by federal subsidies—are cheap to grow, harvest, ship, store, and process. This fiscal advantage over meat, fruits, and vegetables is so compelling that the fact that grains are killing you is conveniently ignored!

If you want to get deep into conspiracy theories, you could explore the fact that high-profit-margin agribiz carbs send lots of customers to high-profit-margin medical-biz hospitals.

To be fair, the reality is that this was not entirely done for profit. Nina Teicholz, author of *The Big Fat Surprise*, argues that she found in her research that:

> On the whole, the mistakes of nutrition science could not primarily be pinned on the nefarious interests of Big Food. The source of our misguided dietary advice was in some ways more disturbing, since it seems to have been driven by experts at some of our most trusted institutions working toward what they believed to be the public good.

Whether intentional or accidental, it's still damaging to our health and wellness. And there's no doubt that this system, which keeps Americans fatter and sicker than anyone else in the developed world, is good for big business. That's why it will continue unless individuals like you get the facts and start to take control of your own diet and health.

## WHAT TO AVOID

Carbohydrates are unhealthy when eaten in large quantities, despite the fact that various versions of the Agriculture Department's food pyramid have instructed us to eat six–11 servings of them per day.

Carbohydrates also hide in unexpected places. Fruit, for example, tends to be rich in carbohydrates. Many advocates of low-carb diets avoid fruits entirely. In my view, fruit can be beneficial, and it includes many of the vitamins and minerals we need. As long as you are eating a healthy diet filled with protein and fat, small amounts of fructose from low-sugar, cold-climate fruits such as berries or apples won't hurt. The carbs to assiduously avoid are the ones in grains, and "whole" grains are generally no better than any others.

The problem with grains is that they are so ubiquitous in the American diet that they have become almost invisible. When the average person goes out for fast food, he worries about the "unhealthy" beef in his 3-ounce-cooked-weight burger and fails to process the fact that the huge bun of quick-digesting grain is the real health-destroyer in the meal. From cereal for breakfast to sandwiches for lunch to pasta for dinner, grains are the centerpiece of every meal—and we pay the price with our health and, ultimately, our lives.

The low-fat health craze also sparked the rise of vegetable oils. Researchers—well intentioned or otherwise—determined that traditional cooking fats like butter and lard were sure to lead to heart disease and should be replaced by "healthier" options like corn, soy, canola, and safflower oils. The truth is vegetable oils are disastrous for your health, particularly when used for deep-frying. When heated, these polyunsaturated oils oxidize, rendering them highly inflammatory—and chronic, elevated, whole-body inflammation underlies a host of diseases ranging from cancers to Alzheimer's to cardiovascular conditions. They also possess an unnatural amount of omega-6 fatty acid, which, even before oxidation, can also be dangerous in high quantities.

As bad as polyunsaturated oils can be, they become even more toxic when they are hydrogenated—that is, transformed into room-temperature solids through an industrial process that adds hydrogen atoms to alter the fat's chemical structure.

In her book *Death by Food Pyramid*, Denise Minger explains how Crisco, one of the first commercial hydrogenated oils, rose to unprecedented popularity just a few years after it was released in 1911.

As Minger puts it:

> Unknown to even the sharpest nutritionists of the day, Crisco
> had invited two killers into the American diet: trans fat result-
> ing from partially hydrogenated oils and an astronomical intake
> of omega-6 fats—both now known to increase the risk of heart
> disease and cause inflammatory immune responses.

To make things worse, the USDA successfully blocked early papers
and research warning against the use of hydrogenated oils. Studies
were even manipulated so that they could be used as citations for the
benefits of vegetable oils when really they increased mortality, cancer
rates, and heart disease.

They were simply too profitable for food manufacturers—far cheaper
to produce than lard, tallow, or butter; tasteless but palatable; and,
because they are relatively inert, a great aid in helping to prolong the
shelf life of baked goods and other processed foods. This happened well
into the 1990s. It wasn't until 2006 that trans fat had to be listed as an
ingredient on labels, and by that time, Americans had been ingesting
them for decades.

## THE LIES ABOUT SATURATED FAT

Google the phrase "artery-clogging saturated fat" and you'll get
back 65,000 results. Pry open the top few hits and you'll find pearls like
"butter contains a lot of artery-clogging saturated fat" and "chicken is
permeated with inherent artery-clogging saturated fat similar to beef."

There's only one minor problem with pronouncements like this:
They are absolutely, categorically false.

The low-sat-fat, high-carb mandate is the most damnable scientific
fraud ever perpetrated on the American public. It's responsible for four
nightmarish decades of spiraling obesity, diabetes, and cancers.

Big Government, Big Food and Big Pharma have brayed this canard for
nearly four decades. Its origins trace back to a 1977 report by Sen. George
McGovern's Select Committee on Nutrition and Human Needs, which featured the phrases "increase carbohydrate consumption" and "reduce
saturated fat consumption." These recommendations were based on
famously cherry-picked data. So right from the start, the science was shaky.

But the directive got traction because it was a gold mine for the industrial food complex. Grain—which yields high-fructose corn syrup and polyunsaturated soybean oil—is dirt-cheap to grow, harvest, process, store, and sell, especially GMO versions cultivated via herbicide-intensive "no-till" agriculture. It's made even cheaper once you throw in all the government subsidies.

This myth also had the extraordinary advantage of sounding sensible. After all, dump a pan of bratwurst grease down your kitchen sink and it forms a clog. Surely, the same logic applies to your arteries too, right?

Wrong. Your body is *optimized* to consume saturated fat. Our ancestors avoided hunting lean animals and gorged on sat-fat from the hump of their dinnertime bison. Meals like that directed their evolution, and we inherited their genes.

Saturated fat, whether from your last meal or your love handles, flows in the bloodstream safely within lipoproteins. And lipoproteins don't randomly "stick" to artery walls. Instead, they adhere in response to inflammation, which is often caused by overeating the aforementioned grains, corn syrup, and seed oils. In the absence of these inflammatory agents, not only are lipoproteins safe, but they can actually remove plaques from arterial walls.

From the start, a few brave researchers argued that the science did not support the anti-sat-fat blather. But it took 33 years for the final word to come out. A huge meta-analysis published in the March 2010 issue of *The American Journal of Clinical Nutrition* found "no significant evidence" that saturated fat in the diet is associated with increased heart disease risk.

Subsequent research has made it clear: The real culprits in raising heart disease risk are sugar, flour, and oxidized seed oils (like the weeks-old soy oil boiling in a fast-food deep fryer). These are what create inflammation, promote obesity, and increase the risk of a wide variety of cancers.

On a practical level, then, this means you should:

- **Eat far less sugar.** In fact, you should cut down on all types of sweeteners. High-fructose corn syrup is neither better nor worse than the rest. Ditch flour-based foods such as breads, cakes, cookies, pancakes, and pretzels. Eschew deep-fried food. It's easier than it sounds. The longer you avoid this junk, the less you desire it

- **Increase your consumption of vegetables.** Go for five–nine servings daily
- **Eat healthful animal-based foods often—at two meals daily at least.** These include pasture-raised beef, pork, chicken, eggs, and wild-caught fish. Also, don't be afraid of organ meats. You should try to eat these twice a month. Did you know calf liver is the most nutrient-dense food you can buy?
- **Eat fruit and nuts,** but sparingly
- **Eat fermented dairy** (cheese, yogurt) if you tolerate it well. Otherwise, skip it
- **Pour your canola, soybean, safflower, and corn oils down the drain.** Use extra virgin olive oil for salads and virgin coconut oil, butter, and nonhydrogenated lard for cooking
- **Put butter in your morning coffee.** This would make most health nuts squirm, I know. However, a tablespoon or so, whirred in the blender, will make your coffee smooth, creamy, and delicious without having to add sugar or over-processed creamers. It also helps to extend your energy boost, rather than making you jittery and come crashing down a few hours later. Also, presenting your body with no carbs and almost pure fat first thing in the morning helps to put you into fat-burning mode for the rest of the day
- For extra credit, **develop a taste for bitter foods such as radicchio and dandelion greens.**

Try alcohol-extracted "bitters" that contain great yellow gentian (Gentiana lutea). Chemicals in these foods moderate blood sugar and optimize digestion. They also cut appetite, helping with weight control.

This is the diet your body—including your arteries—truly needs. You'll be delighted by how it makes you look and feel.

## WEIGHT LOSS BENEFITS

Eating this way can also contribute to weight loss.

One of the earliest diets that led to the observation of this phenomenon was the Atkins diet. By drastically reducing carbohydrates, participants had great results, dropping pounds at a rapid rate. Fascinated by these results, and driven by a shared interest in fitness and nutrition, Drs. Stephen Phinney and Jeff Volek began to look into the biological effects of a low-carb diet in the early 1980s.

They tested athletes like marathon runners, who typically "carbo load" before races to provide them with the fuel they'll need. They found that athletes actually did not require carbohydrates in order to perform their best. In fact, by eliminating carbohydrates as an energy source, our bodies turn to our fat stores for fuel. By removing carbs from our diets, our bodies literally burn fat away.

Weight loss for people on a low-carbohydrate diet is considerably more effective than the standard AHA-recommended diet. Furthermore, the diet has been definitively proved beneficial for heart health. In *The Big Fat Surprise*, Teicholz summarizes the work of Phinney and Volek, saying:

> In trial after trial and by virtually every indicator that they could measure, the high-fat diet was shown to lower the risk for heart disease and diabetes compared to the one low in fat and satu-rated fat that the AHA had proposed to Americans for so long.

Other studies have found that a diet high in fat and low in carbs is also extremely effective against Type 2 diabetes, stabilizing blood glu-cose and insulin levels, due to the absence of carbohydrates.

There are countless other studies detailing how weight loss is often determined more by what you eat than how much you exercise.

One example of this phenomenon is something that plagues many of us—"man boobs." If you're having a hard time losing them no matter how much time you spend in the gym, it could very well be the result of a diet high in estrogen-mimicking compounds, rather than any fault of yours. You can easily remedy this by increasing your intake of estrogen-blocking foods, like cruciferous vegetables (broccoli, cauliflower, Brussels sprouts, kale), mushrooms, and red grapes.

This is just another example of how the foods you eat affect your body more than you may know. Unfortunately, the reason most people have never heard of these facts is not an accident. Corporate food processors, in league with "health" organizations like the American Heart Association and the Academy of Nutrition and Dietetics (both of which get major funding from processed-carb purveyors such as Coca-Cola) do their best to block scientists from publishing any information that goes against their doctrine.

Eric Westman is a doctor and researcher at Duke University. He has performed about a dozen clinical trials on the effects of the Atkins diet. His studies have shown that diets high in fat and low in carbohydrates have unparalleled advantages in the fight against obesity, heart disease, blood pressure, and diabetes. Despite the evidence, he and his team have a very hard time getting published in science journals or being invited to speak at conferences. He is convinced that this is a result of the existing bias in the media, public conscience, and nutrition community. Teicholz quotes him as saying:

> When an unscientific fear of dietary fat pervades the culture so much that the researchers who are on study sections that provide funding will not allow research into high-fat diets for fear of "harming people," this situation will not allow science to "self-correct." A sort of scientific taboo is created because of the low likelihood of funding.

Not only are these government-backed institutions prescribing us the wrong diets, but they're also actively impeding the truth about nutrition from reaching the American people.

Read on to discover how you can stop this cycle of lies in its tracks.

## BEEF—THE NEW SUPERFOOD

We've already covered how and why red meat came to have such a negative connotation in our country. Claims that it raises your cholesterol, clogs your arteries, and increases your risk of heart disease have caused many people to abandon red meats for leaner options like chicken and fish.

The truth is, however, the muscles and organs of cattle are packed with nutrients that you won't be able to get from the alternatives.

Steak actually has several nutritional advantages over chicken. It is high in iron, zinc, potassium, and vitamin B-12. In fact, a 3-ounce serving of sirloin steak contains 1.6 milligrams of iron, which is essential for brain development and immune function, as well as 4.5 milligrams of zinc, which allows you to taste, smell, and also improve immune function. Comparatively, the same-sized serving of chicken contains only 0.9 milligrams of each of these elements.[1]

Vitamin B-12 promotes brain function and the formation of red blood cells. Animal products are the only reliable source, but a serving of sirloin steak provides 1.5 micrograms, whereas chicken only has 0.3 micrograms.

You also shouldn't forget about the organs. Although they've been largely abandoned on our menus, ingredients like liver, sweetbreads, brains, kidneys, tendons, and bones were all featured in our cookbooks for generations and were highly valued for their nutrition content in many cultures.

Both red meat and liver contain more iron, vitamins, potassium, magnesium, and other nutrients than carrots or apples do. In fact, ounce for ounce, beef liver has eight times the vitamin C of apples and 50 times the vitamin A of carrots. Just take a look at the chart on the following page for more comparisons.

---

1 "Health Advantage of Beef Over Chicken." SF Gate. Web.

| | Apple (100 g) | Carrots (100 g) | Red Meat (100 g) | Beef Liver (100 g) |
|---|---|---|---|---|
| Calcium | 3.0 mg | 3.3 mg | 11.0 mg | 11.0 mg |
| Phosphorus | 6.0 mg | 31.0mg | 140.0 mg | 476.0 mg |
| Magnesium | 4.8 mg | 6.2 mg | 15.0 mg | 18.0 mg |
| Potassium | 139.0 mg | 222.0 mg | 370.0 mg | 380.0 mg |
| Iron | .1 mg | .6 mg | 3.3 mg | 8.8 mg |
| Zinc | .05 mg | .3 mg | 4.4 mg | 4.0 mg |
| Copper | .04 mg | .08 mg | .18 mg | 12.0 mg |
| Vitamin A | None | None | 40 IU | 53,500 IU |
| Vitamin D | None | None | Trace | 19 IU |
| Vitamin E | .37 mg | .11 mg | 1.7 mg | .63mg |
| Vitamin C | 7.0 mg | 6.0 mg | None | 27.0 mg |
| Thiamin | .03 mg | .05 mg | .05 mg | .26 mg |
| Riboflavin | .02 mg | .05 mg | .20 mg | 4.19 mg |
| Niacin | .10 mg | .60 mg | 4.0 mg | 16.5 mg |
| Pantothenic Acid | .11 mg | .19 mg | .4 mg | 8.8 mg |
| Vitamin B6 | .03 mg | .10 mg | .07 mg | .73 mg |
| Folic Acid | 8.0 mcg | 24.0 mcg | 4.0 mcg | 145.0 mcg |
| Biotin | None | .42 mcg | 2.08 mcg | 96.0 mcg |
| Vitamin B12 | None | None | 1.84 mcg | 111.3 mcg |

Source: Chris Kresser

# EAT THIS, DON'T EAT THAT

How often do you find yourself staring at a menu wondering what you should choose?

You might really *want* to order a mouthwatering rack of ribs and an ice-cold pint of beer. I know I do.

But the little voice in the back of your head—or, let's be honest, your spouse's voice from over your shoulder—encourages you to pick the healthy option.

Is there anything more frustrating than denying yourself the foods you want and not seeing any results?

As I've said before, this is simply not your fault.

It may surprise you that the meals you've been considering healthy options are actually worse for you in the long run. In some cases, the foods you're longing to eat are the better choice, even if you're being told the opposite.

Below are a few examples of how the dominant ideas of what's good versus bad to eat might not be correct after all. Sometimes, the rich foods you crave are better after all!

## LOW-FAT YOGURT AND FRUIT *OR* BACON AND CHEDDAR OMELET?

Most people would assume that sticking to a yogurt mixed with fruit for breakfast is the way to go. However, you might want to think twice about how to begin your day.

To create low-fat products like yogurt, manufacturers have to take the fat out and put something else in—usually sugar. A fat-free "healthy" yogurt can have just as much sugar in it as a Snickers bar!

As an Op-Ed by Teicholz in *The Wall Street Journal* points out, "Even seemingly healthy low-fat foods, such as yogurt, are stealth carb-delivery systems, since removing the fat often requires the addition of fillers to make up for lost texture—and these are usually carbohydrate-based."[2]

The carbohydrates and sugar in your fruit and yogurt make insulin spike, which means stored fat. It also means hitting that midmorning slump and often being hungry again by 10 a.m.

Eggs, in comparison, are high in protein and good fats, containing the essential amino acids our bodies need for growth and repair.

Bacon and whole-fat cheese, when sourced from grass-fed animals free of hormones, are nothing but beneficial for you.

It wasn't until Americans started replacing animal fats with carbohydrates and vegetable oils that we really saw the rise of coronary disease. So throw in some sautéed, nutrient-dense organic vegetables and eat your omelet—and cook it in clarified butter, too!

## WHOLE WHEAT VEGGIE SANDWICH *OR* PORK CHOP WITH GRAVY AND LEAFY GREENS?

Go for the pork. Pork supplies essential protein and fat, while the greens provide vital nutrients, and neither of them will spike your insulin like grain-based carbohydrates.

Excessive carbohydrates lead not only to obesity but also over time to Type 2 diabetes and heart disease. And bread supplies one of the biggest carb loads of all.

It's not just white flour that's the problem. Even though we are told that whole wheat bread is a healthy choice, Teicholz suggests even that can do harm:

Too much whole-grain oatmeal for breakfast and whole-grain pasta for dinner, with fruit snacks in between, add up to a less healthy diet than one of eggs and bacon, followed by fish.

2 "The Questionable Link Between Saturated Fat and Heart Disease." The Wall Street Journal. Web.

The reality is that fat doesn't make you fat or diabetic. Scientific investigations going back to the 1950s suggest that, actually, carbs do.[3]

Meanwhile, greens like kale, chard, spinach, and collards provide vitamins and minerals that are otherwise hard to obtain, like magnesium, potassium, calcium, and manganese.[4] Consuming them will help protect you against disease, promote heart health, and stimulate your brain.

They are also rich in fiber, which can "lower cholesterol and blood pressure, and help to temper blood sugar swings by slowing the absorption of carbohydrates into your bloodstream after meals."[5]

Swapping out your midday sandwich for a nice piece of meat and a salad drizzled with quality extra virgin olive oil won't just taste great. It will nourish you and help give you the energy you need for the rest of your day.

## PLATE OF HUMMUS AND PITA *OR* BISON BURGER WITH AVOCADO AND CHEESE?

Hummus and pita are high in carbs, while avocados, bison meat, and full-fat cheese offer healthy fats and keep insulin low and steady. Snacking on hummus and pita chips will curb your hunger for a short amount of time but provide you with very little nutritional value. Once your body comes down from the insulin spike of those chips, you'll be hungry again.

What you should aim for is to eat a meal that is nutrient-packed and provides you with other dietary benefits. That way, you won't only satisfy your hunger, but also feed your body and mind.

The National Bison Association cites research that shows that the "meat from bison is a highly nutrient-dense food because of the proportion of protein, fat, mineral, and fatty acids to its caloric value . . . Bison has a greater concentration of iron as well as some of the essential fatty acids necessary for human well-being."[6]

---

3 "The Questionable Link Between Saturated Fat and Heart Disease." The Wall Street Journal. Web.

4 "Why You Should Eat Leafy Greens." Mark's Daily Apple. Web.

5 "Leafy Green Vegetables: How Food Affects Health." Joy Bauer. Web.

6 "Nutritional Information." National Bison Association. Web.

Avocados have also long been heralded as a superfood. They're high in healthy fats called oleic acid—the same found in olive oil. Oleic acid has been linked to reduced inflammation and has beneficial effects on genes linked to a lowered risk of cancer. They also are high in antioxidants and fiber.

Ounce for ounce, avocados also contain more potassium than a banana, with a 100 grams per serving. Authoritynutrition.com has several studies listed that "show that having a high potassium intake is linked to reduced blood pressure, a major risk factor for heart attacks, strokes, and kidney failure."[7]

Best of all, they're delicious!

Combining bison meat, avocado, and some full-fat cheese together makes for a lunch that is more filling and more nutritious than an empty snack of hummus and pita chips. You can add other veggies as toppings as well, if you'd like.

Just make sure that you skip the bun!

And as we've seen, these fats are not harmful. Even famed TV doctor Mehmet Oz admitted he was wrong about fats.

After promoting a low-fat diet for years, he make a shocking admission to his audience: "For years I have warned you about the health risks of a diet high in saturated fat," said Dr. Oz. "Today I'm coming to a shocking realization; 40 years of diet advice may be completely wrong! In a revolutionary reversal, more doctors, including myself, are saying that saturated fat may not be so bad for you after all."[8]

## STEAK AND BROCCOLI *OR* CHICKEN CAESAR SALAD?

Steak and broccoli is the winner here. Steak is full of good saturated fats, including one called stearic acid that may actually lower heart disease risk, and broccoli provides a range of healthful micronutrients.

Although chicken is often touted as being the healthier choice, that is largely because it is low in fat. We've already put the two head-to-head in this report and have shown how steak is higher in many nutrients.

---

7 "12 Proven Benefits of Avocado." Authority Nutrition. Web.

8 "The Truth About Saturated Fat." Dr. Oz. Web.

The croutons and Caesar dressing involved in a chicken Caesar salad are empty carbohydrates. And although romaine lettuce is comparable to broccoli in regard to nutritional value, containing antioxidants, protein, magnesium, and calcium, being smothered in Caesar dressing pretty much eliminates those benefits.

An average serving of Caesar dressing has about 1,200 calories, 7 g of sugars, and an astonishing 2,533 mg of sodium—that's 106% of the suggested daily value, in case you were wondering.

Remember, dietary fat doesn't mean fat on your body, and dietary cholesterol doesn't mean cholesterol in your blood. Your liver makes most of the cholesterol—an absolutely vital organic compound—that your body needs. Eating cholesterol simply spares your liver the burden of synthesizing so much of this essential compound.

And as Nina Teicholz says, animal foods like red meat, milk, cheese, and eggs "are particularly dense in nutrients—far more so that fruits and vegetables. They contain fat and protein in the proportion that humans need. They have been shown to provide the best possible nutrition for healthy growth and reproduction."

Never assume that a salad is going to be the healthiest choice on your menu. In many cases, a well-balanced entree will provide more nutritional value.

## SWEET POTATO WEDGES *OR* MASHED POTATOES?

Go for sweet potatoes every time.

Normally, potatoes are something we'd suggest you avoid, since they are high in starch and other carbohydrates. They cause your blood pressure to spike and then dramatically fall.

However, potatoes make up a huge part of our diets. French fries, mashed potatoes, baked potatoes with bacon and sour cream—we crave them all.

Sweet potatoes are a great compromise if you're looking to supplement that part of your meal with something a little healthier.

Sweet potatoes offer not only delectable taste, but also two big health advantages over the common white potato—a 58% lower glycemic index (a measure of a food's ability to raise blood sugar) and far higher nutrient density. Sweet potatoes are especially rich in beta carotene, which the body converts to vitamin A.

They're also delicious, which always helps!

## GLASS OF RED WINE *OR* GREEN SMOOTHIE?

This one's a little different. A green smoothie is full of vitamins and minerals and could very well be a healthy part of your day.

But which would you really prefer?

The truth is there are a ton of benefits to moderate drinking. And when you put a fine wine next to a smoothie that looks suspiciously like baby food, I think we both know what you'd like to choose.

Some reports show that drinking one glass of wine is equal to one hour of exercise.

The secret is resveratrol, which improves physical performance, heart function, and muscle strength.

The study came out of the University of Alberta. Principal investigator Jason Dyck said that he and his team "were excited when [they] saw that resveratrol showed results similar to what you would see from extensive endurance exercise training."[9]

Reports from Harvard also now confirm that "red wine may contain more and more various substances in addition to alcohol that could prevent blood clots, relax blood vessel walls, and prevent the oxidation of low-density lipoprotein (LDL, 'bad' cholesterol), a key early step in the formation of cholesterol-filled plaque."[10]

Overall, you should be able to indulge in any alcoholic beverage with dinner. Harvard's report also shows that in a study of 38,000 men over 12 years, "moderate drinkers were 30–35% less likely to have had a heart attack than nondrinkers." This benefit came regardless of drinking beer, wine, or spirits.

---

9 "Resveratrol may be natural exercise performance enhancer." Science Daily. Web.

10 "Is Wine Fine, or Beer Better?" Harvard School of Public Health. Web.

## DARK CHOCOLATE BAR *OR* STRAWBERRY SHORTCAKE?

Go for the chocolate!

Dark chocolate is a great source of antioxidants and minerals. A 100-gram bar of dark chocolate can provide almost your entire daily dose of manganese as well as almost 70% of the iron you need in a day.

There are also clinical trials showing correlations between cocoa and lower blood pressure as well as lowering the risk for heart disease. Some studies have also shown cocoa powder to lower the amount of "bad" LDL cholesterol while increasing levels of "good" HDL.

Other theories suggest that chocolate releases feel-good hormones like dopamine and serotonin in your brain. It can satisfy your sweet tooth and add a delicious bit of diversification to your diet.

Despite the strawberries on top, shortcake is filled with carbs and sugar that you don't need to enjoy dessert. Keep it simple and go for dark chocolate.

# FREEDOM FROM COUNTING CALORIES:
## Keep Track of *These* to Burn Maximum Fat Instead

Forget counting calories to burn fat.

It's a pain in the butt.

Few people will even bother to start.

Even *fewer* people will keep going long term.

And one more minor detail—it doesn't work—or at least it doesn't work for most of us. If you've tried calorie restriction in the past and it failed for you, you're not alone.

*In fact, it's failed us as a country:* Nationwide data shows that even though we're eating fewer calories than we did roughly 10 years ago, we're getting fatter.[11]

Keep that in mind the next time anyone tries to tell you burning fat is a simple matter of dropping your calorie intake. Personally, I think this data should be memorized by every doctor who ever sees an overweight patient struggling with sticking to a low-calorie diet. And if they forget, they must write on a chalkboard (in cursive!) "I will not recommend low-calorie diets to patients who want to lose weight" a hundred times.

Allow me to get back on track here with some very good news. Science has shown there's a certain trick you can use to lose weight without restricting calories at all. In other words, you can eat until you're fully satisfied and (as long as you're not stuffing yourself) you will burn fat.

---

11 "Trends in energy intake among adults in the United States: Findings from NHANES." The American Journal of Clinical Nutrition. Web.

In fact, a study out of the University of Cincinnati and Children's Hospital Medical Center showed using this trick can help you lose more than twice as much weight and burn more than twice as much fat than if you exert massive willpower to drop your calorie consumption. [12]

But the benefits don't end there. Take a gander at these and see which appeals most to you:

- Appetite regulation: You'll feel more full, with fewer blood sugar spikes and dips that lead to intense hunger and cravings
- Enhanced focus and mental clarity
- More energy
- Lower blood sugar and insulin levels
- Increased HDL ("good") cholesterol
- Lower triglycerides
- Effective seizure control (it has been used for this since the '30s)
- Enhanced athletic performance
- Reduced inflammation, which may lower risk of—or reduce, arrest, or reverse progression of—a wide variety of conditions including:
  - Alzheimer's disease
  - Cancers, including late-stage cancers
  - Cardiovascular disease
  - Parkinson's disease
  - Type 2 diabetes
  - Polycystic ovarian syndrome.

Enough buildup. What is this trick?

It's pretty simple. Instead of counting calories, count the number of carbohydrate grams you eat. More specifically, keep them low. Way low. As in, under 60 grams per day, maximum.

A tall order for most people, but the science shows this is as close to a surefire method to flip your fat-burning switch on as you're ever going to get this side of liposuction.

---

12 "A Randomized Trial Comparing a Very Low Carbohydrate Diet and a Calorie-Restricted Low Fat Diet on Body Weight and Cardiovascular Risk Factors in Healthy Women." The Journal of Clinical Endocrinology & Metabolism. Web.

Here's how it works:

When your body doesn't have carbohydrates for fuel, your liver and kidneys begin to metabolize fats. As a result, special compounds called ketones are produced. Then they're delivered to your cells where they're used to make adenosine triphosphate, known—mercifully—by the abbreviation ATP.

Your body uses ATP for energy. In other words, this entire chemical process is how your body quite literally *burns fat for fuel*.

The "catch" is your body will not do this as long as there's enough glucose in your muscles, liver, and blood for easy energy.

So you must do two things:

1. Swear off eating more than 60 grams of carbs per day.
2. Weather the adjustment process as your body switches to burning its fat stores for fuel, which usually takes around two weeks.

It's a shame, but most people don't last more than two or three weeks on a low-carb diet, which means they tend to quit precisely when the true fat-burning effects start kicking in.

If you're still on the fence about trying to cut carbs (or attempting to cut them again), keep this in mind: It'll be much easier now that you know (if you read **Sin Foods For Your Health** prior to this chapter) you *can* eat liberal amounts of saturated fat in the form of meat and butter.

Let's be honest: Is it really so hard to skip the bread if you know you can splurge on a juicy steak instead? With a pat of butter on top?

However, I understand you may still have some reservations about trying this trick. Especially if you've attempted a very low carbohydrate approach before and it didn't turn out like you'd hoped.

First, as I've mentioned, ditching the sugar, grains, and other carbohydrate concoctions can be nigh impossible when you're under the impression you have to eat like a politically correct bird. But you don't. Natural fats are back on the menu. Enjoy them and the satiety they provide.

Second, you have to be more nuanced than usual in your approach to very low carb if you want to succeed long term. Most people can't make it past the first couple weeks, which is your body's adjustment period. This is the "make or break" transition when your body ditches burning sugar for fuel . . . and switches to burning body fat.

These first two weeks might not be pleasant. Some side effects include:

- Constipation/diarrhea (MCT oil like coconut oil can have a laxative effect, so start with small amounts!)
- Fatigue and headaches
- Muscle cramping due to water loss (eating more salt, drinking bouillon, and taking magnesium can help with this)
- Increased risk for kidney stones (again, always make sure you drink plenty of water).

Another disadvantage of this strategy is that it's inconvenient—at least at first. Most restaurant meals fall out of bounds, unless it's a strict meat-and-veggie combo. And prepackaged, store-bought foods are an absolute nightmare of processed carbs, minimized fat, unhealthy preservatives, and addictive artificial flavorings to keep you coming back for more.

But if you can withstand temptation and muster your willpower . . . fat-burning success doesn't get simpler than this.

## STEPS TO FREEDOM

1. Eat fewer carbs, until you're consuming a maximum of 60 grams per day.
2. When in doubt, see Step 1.

In all seriousness, here's a general breakdown of what your daily fat-protein-carb ratio should be:

60–70% fat

20–30% protein

0–10% carbohydrate

The more you can make a game out of avoiding carbs, especially from processed and grain sources, the greater your chances of winning the fat-loss battle.

This is especially vital in the morning. Big Grain has done a bang-up job brainwashing the American public into believing a hefty helping of cereal and bagels every morning (with sweet orange juice, which is metabolically identical to soda!) is the way to start your day off right. And they have a point—it will give you plenty of quick energy.

What they don't mention is if you want to burn fat, your body should **not** have a massive injection of easy-to-process energy stores first thing every morning. Otherwise . . . why would it bother making ketones out of body fat?

By avoiding carbs, especially in the morning, you force your body to rapidly deplete its reserves of glucose. Once they're exhausted, ketosis begins and your fat gets burned.

Because this is such a charged, controversial subject, you might still have some questions. Indeed, probably one of the most common reasons people abandon otherwise-effective low-carb diets is because well-meaning but misguided friends scare and shame them into returning to "heart-healthy whole grains."

So here's some reassurance of what the science says, in case you have your doubts:

**Question:** *I've read about/experienced low-carb diets causing headaches and fatigue. Doesn't that mean they're bad?*

**Answer:** The vast majority of the time, it simply means you're excreting more water and salt than usual. The solution is just as basic:

Drink more water.

Eat more salt.

Concerned about the health effects of the latter? Don't be. First of all, you're excreting more salt through your urine anyway, so eating more in response won't increase your net amount. Plus, new research is showing the whole connection between salt intake and heart health is much more complicated than we originally thought . . . and natural salt isn't so bad after all (honestly, does this even surprise you?).[13]

**Question:** *I'm eating more natural fats now, so why is my weight loss stalled?*

**Answer:** It's not enough to simply eat more fat. Frankly, who wouldn't want to add more fat to a high-carb diet? Pardon me, waiter, I'll have another hot-fudge sundae!

---

13 "The wrong white crystals: not salt but sugar as aetiological in hypertension and cardiometabolic disease." Open Heart. Web.

You must combine adding more fat (the easy part) with eating less than 60 grams of carbohydrate per day (the hard part). The only solace I can offer is that it gets easier over time. Within a month, you'll find the concept of pounding down the U.S. average of 350–500 grams of carbs daily rather disgusting—sort of like idea of drinking a big glass of maple syrup.

**Question:** *Should I eat high amounts of protein?*

**Answer:** This is an excellent question. And if you've ever tried the low-carb diet approach and it didn't work for you, *high* levels of protein may have been why. That's not a typo.

Your liver can convert protein to glucose (a form of sugar you can use as fuel) through a process called gluconeogenesis. If this occurs, ketosis cannot be achieved, and your fat-burning switch doesn't flip on.

As counterintuitive as it sounds, in order to maximize your fat-burning potential, you need to eat a **high-fat,** *moderate-to-low-protein,* **low-carb diet.**

No wonder so many people are overweight today. This is almost exactly the opposite of the ratios recommended by the government and official "health" associations such as the American Heart Association. It's also the opposite of the most common foods you'll find in the grocery store.

**Question:** *I heard all the weight lost on a low-carb diet is just water weight.*

**Answer:** Like some pervasive rumors, this falsehood began with a grain of truth. When you first cut carbs, you will lose more water (which is why you must drink more water to compensate, or you might feel sluggish and get headaches).

This is because each gram of blood sugar is dissolved in about four grams water. So as you burn the stored sugar, the water that holds it in solution gets excreted as well. So you can rapidly lose weight immediately after switching to a low-carb diet . . . and rapidly gain it back if you "cheat" and have some carbs.

This has nothing to do with fat loss—it's just that rising and falling sugar levels cause the amount of water in your blood, muscles, and liver to fluctuate dramatically.

Just stick with the low-carb regimen. Once the water weight is expelled, you'll start burning fat. You'll keep losing weight, but it will happen more slowly.

**Question:** *But what about all the vitamins and minerals in fruits? They have plenty of carbs, but don't I need them to survive and be healthy?*

**Answer:** Absolutely not. No one needs fruit to be healthy. There is not a single vitamin or mineral in fruit that cannot be obtained more abundantly in vegetables, not to mention in organ meats (beef liver, for example, has four times as much vitamin C per gram as an apple). The whole "fruits and vegetables are vital" mantra, repeated endlessly by every mainstream nutrition "expert," has convinced most Americans that these two classes of food are equally healthful. That's absolutely false. Low-sugar vegetables—especially the leafy greens—are vastly superior to fruits for overall health.

**Question:** *I heard that ketosis is a dangerous medical condition!*

**Answer:** You probably heard this about *ketoacidosis*, which is very different from ketosis. Ketoacidosis is a dangerous buildup of ketones in the blood. They're acidic, so too many ketone bodies acidify the blood, which can lead to serious effects. Ketoacidosis occurs when ketones levels are high *and* blood sugar levels are high as well because the pancreas isn't properly producing insulin. It's a potential concern only for Type 1 diabetics who cannot produce insulin.

Another important point: A natural ketogenic diet can produce fantastic results for someone suffering from Type 2 diabetes. Most of these people still have the potential to produce insulin but aren't able to regulate their levels because of their lifestyle and diet. For these folks, a ketogenic diet might eliminate their diabetes altogether.

# EXCEPTIONAL FAT-BURNING FOODS

I roll my eyes whenever some "expert" blithely recites the mainstream weight-loss mantra: "Losing weight is just a matter of calories in and calories out."

This simple sentence aggravates me for two reasons:

1. Most men and women care about a lot more than merely losing weight: It's also the *composition* of said lost weight that matters, as well as how easily it's dropped.
2. Oh, and the phrase is <u>wrong</u>.

You see, calories are an old, discredited measure of the "fattening" potential of a food. Most people don't know that the whole concept of calories was borrowed from steam-engine designers.

They invented it in the 1810s and 1820s to help them determine which fuel would make an engine run longest. Nutrition "scientists" borrowed it in the 1870s to help them discover which food would "fuel" laborers most cheaply.

The problem? Human beings are not steam engines. We don't "burn" foods. We metabolize them in complex ways that make calories a crude, inaccurate measure of how much energy—or fat—we can make from them.

Consequently, two foods with *identical* calorie counts can have dramatically *different* effects on our fat cells.

As you'll read below, certain foods have been shown through scientific studies to cause an *exceptional* amount of fat-burning.

Don't get me wrong: The foundation of your fat loss will come from the broad, general principles laid out in **Freedom From Fat**. No amount of special ingredients will make up for the high-carb, low-fat nonsense supported by most nutritional gurus and our government.

But if you want every advantage on your side for exceptional fat burning, then the science indicates these foods can help.

## GREEN TEA

Green tea is a "superfood." Its many health benefits have earned it an important place in diets worldwide, particularly as an integral part of Eastern food and medicine.

The studies on green tea's powers for weight loss are overwhelming. The secret lies in something called "catechins." Catechins are tannins found in green tea that provide powerful antioxidant activity—they're essentially green tea's "active ingredient."

One study monitored 182 moderately overweight Chinese subjects to see the effects of catechin in green tea.[14] Researchers concluded that two servings of extra-high catechin green tea per day reduced total body fat, body composition, and abdominal fatness.

When consumed every day, and combined with exercise three times a week, green tea with catechins was found to enhance "exercise-induced changes in abdominal fat," showing that green tea could help accelerate the results of exercise.[15]

(Normally, this would be the appropriate time for me to crank up the font size and declare: "Green Tea Blasts Away Belly Fat!" but you've already gotten your hands on these guides, so I don't think you need to be beaten over the head with the benefits of this amazing beverage.)

Moreover, the University of Birmingham's School of Sport and Exercise Sciences found that consuming green tea extract "can increase fat

---

14 "Effects of catechin enriched green tea on body composition." Obesity. Web.

15 "Green tea catechin consumption enhances exercise-induced abdominal fat loss in overweight and obese adults." The Journal of Nutrition. Web.

oxidation during moderate-intensity exercise and can improve insulin sensitivity and glucose tolerance in healthy young men."[16] The benefits have been seen in both obese and healthy participants.

It's also better for weight loss than just drinking coffee or black tea. One meta-analysis out of the Department of Human Biology, Nutrition and Toxicology Research Institute at Maastricht University set out to find whether catechin-caffeine mixtures (like green tea) were more effective in increasing energy expenditure and weight loss than caffeine on its own.[17]

Researchers evaluated six similar, high-quality studies and found that while both caffeine and catechin-caffeine mixtures boosted energy expenditure, only the catechin-caffeine mixture (green tea) contributed to fat oxidation—in other words, a loss of body fat.

Take a page out of the book of Chinese medicine and add green tea to your daily routine. That, combined with some healthy exercise, will accelerate your weight loss.

## GRAPEFRUIT

This pucker-inducing tangy fruit also has hidden weight-loss power.

Researchers from the Department of Nutrition and Metabolic Research at Scripps Clinic in La Jolla, California, put grapefruit to the test against apple juice and asked 91 obese patients to include variations of fresh grapefruit, grapefruit juice, apple juice, or a placebo before each of their three daily meals.[18]

In the end, "the fresh grapefruit group lost significantly more weight than the placebo group," and the weight loss benefits for a fresh grapefruit also beat out the juice alternatives.

Grapefruit consumption also resulted in "modest weight loss . . . a significant reduction in waist circumference . . . and a significant reduction in systolic blood pressure." Although the researchers from

---

16 "Green tea extract ingestion, fat oxidation, and glucose tolerance in healthy humans." The American Journal of Clinical Nutrition. Web.

17 "The effects of catechin rich teas and caffeine on energy expenditure and fat oxidation: a meta-analysis." Obesity Reviews. Web.

18 "The effects of grapefruit on weight and insulin resistance: relationship to the metabolic syndrome." Journal of Medicinal Food. Web.

that particular study were not able to conclude that it significantly decreased body weight, they determined that the "improvements in blood pressure and lipids demonstrated in the intervention group suggest that grapefruit should be further evaluated in the context of obesity and cardiovascular disease prevention."[19]

Based on these results, choose a little grapefruit instead of <u>any</u> kind of grain and make it one of your first choices of fruit.

## SPINACH

You remember Popeye, don't you? The rough-and-tough sailor who could pump up his arms at will by downing a can of spinach, usually to save his damsel-girlfriend Olive Oyl.

Turns out he might have been on to something. A recent study from Lund University in Sweden published in the journal *Appetite* followed 38 women for 12 weeks.[20] Scientists asked them to add a special extract from spinach leaves to their diet in the form of a green smoothie at breakfast. The women were also asked to eat three meals and exercise for 30 minutes daily.

Result? The extract induced weight loss. Furthermore, it lessened the urge for sweets and fat, curbing appetite, from the first day of the study through the last. Women following the regimen lost an average of 11 pounds!

These extracts are green-plant membranes called thylakoids, which slow down the digestive process, allowing you to feel more full and satisfied after a meal. The scientists in this study theorize that thylakoids also reduce cravings for sweets.

One woman who participated in the experiment admitted she used to feel food cravings, especially in the evening. But when she added a shot of thylakoids to her diet, she said, "I didn't have those cravings at all. They disappeared."[21]

---

19 "The effects of daily consumption of grapefruit on body weight, lipids, and blood pressure in healthy, overweight adults." Metabolism. Web.

20 "Body weight loss, reduced urge for palatable food and increased release of GLP-1 through daily supplementation with green-plant membranes for three months in overweight women". Appetite. Web.

21 "Spinach extract curbs appetite, sugar cravings". YouTube, Lund University. Web.

Green-plant membranes are found in all green plants, but we're focusing on spinach because it's so versatile. While it's a great healthy option anytime, for fat loss, I suggest you consume it just as the participants did in the study:

Grind some spinach in a blender with water, so the thylakoids are freed from the plant cells, and take a shot before your first meal of the day. Add some hard liquor if that helps it go down. (I'm only kidding . . . sort of.)

## HOT PEPPERS

First, let me introduce you to something called capsaicin—a component of chili peppers. Capsaicin is the stuff that makes your eyes burn if you happen to rub them after chopping a jalapeno.

If this has never happened to you, take it from me—it's not a pleasant experience.

Capsaicin creates a burning sensation when it contacts skin or eyes or is ingested. It's what makes many spicy foods so intense.

Although capsaicin acts as an irritant for humans on an external level, recent studies have shown that peppers rich in the stuff could accelerate weight loss.

One study evaluated 10 men, giving them capsaicin an hour before low-intensity exercise.[22] (The participants were given a coated tablet, so they avoided the spicy-taste side effects.)

The researchers found that capsaicin "is a valuable supplement for the treatment of individuals with hyperlipidemia and/or obesity because it improves lipolysis without any adverse effects on the cardiac depolarization and repolarization process."

In English, this means it can help break down fats without the negative side effect of speeding up heart rate. Ingesting capsaicin has also been shown to decrease appetite and increase satiety—you'll feel the need to eat less often and feel more satisfied when you do.

---

22 "Alterations of autonomic nervous activity and energy metabolism by capsaicin ingestion during aerobic exercise in healthy men." Journal of nutritional science and vitaminology. Web.

Researchers from the Oxford Polytechnic Institute found a "diet-induced thermic effect" resulting from participants adding chiles and hot mustard to their meals.[23]

By adding three grams of chilies and three grams of hot mustard to their meals, the volunteers in the study increased their metabolism by 25%.

According to George Harris, then editor-in-chief of American Health, "What the Oxford researchers have discovered is that hot peppers raise the thermic effect 25% higher than the normal jump, about 45 calories per 700 (consumed). Now, that's not a huge effect and it's not going to make us all become pepper dieters. But if you combine it with other healthy eating habits, you've got a major prospect."

The long-term effects have not been proven. Eventually, most people do build up a resistance to spicy foods and might not continue to see the same results.

But if you're not used to spicy food, and want to give your metabolism a little extra kick, adding some hot pepper sauce and hot mustard to your meal might just do the trick.

## VITAMIN D

Vitamin D is good for more than just building strong bones.

A double-blind randomized clinical trial observed the effects of vitamin D3 supplements at a dosage of 1,000 IU daily on 77 healthy, overweight, and obese women.[24] They found that the supplements resulted in body fat mass reduction.

Research has shown that having low vitamin D levels makes you more likely to be overweight, with less muscle mass and more belly fat.[25] Having low levels of vitamin D increases fat storage in the body, slowing metabolism.

This is true of men and women of all ages and ethnicities. Adding vitamin D to your diet could help you shed those extra pounds without altering your diet or exercise routines. An estimated 75% of American

---

23 "Feel The Burn The Hottest News: Chilies Speed Up Metabolism And Eat Into Calories." Sun Sentinel. Web.

24 "A 12-week double-blind randomized clinical trial of vitamin D3 supplementation on body fat mass in healthy overweight and obese women." Nutrition journal. Web.

25 "Optimize Your Vitamin D Level To Lose Fat & Gain Muscle". Poliquin Group. Web.

teens and adults are deficient in this vital nutrient—which means you probably are as well.

## COCONUT OIL

For all the nutritional faux experts out there who still blather that "a calorie is a calorie" when it comes to fat loss, I'd like to introduce them to coconut oil.

Specifically, the fat that's abundant in coconuts, called medium chain triglycerides—or MCTs, for short.

Your body metabolizes this kind of fat differently from others, taking it to the liver for immediate energy use.

One study set out to test how effective MCT supplements would be for enhancing fat loss in a low-calorie diet.[26] Obese women were observed for four weeks, and the group of women taking MCT supplements "showed a significantly greater decrease in body weight during the first two weeks." They also experienced less hunger and more satiety—the feeling of fullness—after meals. These differences gradually decreased after the first two weeks but never disappeared.

Another study from the School of Dietetics and Human Nutrition at McGill University studied young, healthy women and found that MCT was able to "increase endogenous oxidation of long-chain saturated fatty acids."[27] In other words, it boosted the body's ability to burn all types of fat, which suggested MCT would be able to play a role in body weight control long term.

A 2003 study showed that not only is the fat found in coconut oil highly thermogenic—eating it tends to increase energy expenditure (fat burning) compared against the same amount of calories from other fats—but it can also help you lose more weight.[28]

Still another found it shrinks the dreaded belly fat.

---

26 "Value of VLCD supplementation with medium chain triglycerides." PubMed. Web.

27 "Endogenous fat oxidation during medium chain versus long chain triglyceride feeding in healthy women." International Journal of Obesity and Related Metabolic Disorders. Web.

28 "Greater rise in fat oxidation with medium-chain triglyceride consumption relative to long-chain triglyceride is associated with lower initial body weight and greater loss of subcutaneous adipose tissue." International Journal of Obesity and Related Metabolic Disorders. Web.

Paging through all the science on coconut oil's health-promoting and fat-burning effects is no easy task. But luckily for you, coconut oil is easy to add to your diet.

Simply replace "vegetable oil" (the marketing moniker for soybean oil) with coconut oil—it's better for you and will help jump-start your weight loss. If you like the taste, grab a spoonful whenever you have a craving for food.

Try it on your skin, too! You might be pleasantly surprised.

## RED MEAT

Eat healthy animal-based foods. For over 50 years, animal-based foods have been demonized in the U.S. as contributors to elevated risk of heart disease. Even today, the vegan diet—devoid of all animal-derived foods, including meat, milk, and eggs—is held by many to be the gold standard in healthy eating.

None of this makes any sense. Studies have only been able to show an association between red meat and chronic health problems because the only people who consumed it in quantity were those who ignored all health advice—in other words, they also smoked, were sedentary, ate copious amounts of processed carbohydrates, and so on.

Studies that link beef consumption to cancer, diabetes, and so on are invariably tainted by these "confounding" variables. Further, no large-scale study I've been able to locate has bothered to differentiate between health effects of eating beef from grain-fed versus grass-fed cattle—despite the fact that grass-fed animals have a more favorable ratio of heart-healthy omega-3 fats.

And yet even without this important distinction, a 2014 report in the journal Meat Science explains that "large population studies both in Europe and North America have recently reported no association between intakes of unprocessed red meat and any cause of death, including cardiovascular disease or cancer."[29]

Red meat and other animal proteins are a healthy, necessary part of the human diet. We went into more detail in the *"Sin Foods for*

---

29 "Red meats: Time for a paradigm shift in dietary advice." Meat Science. Web.

*Healthy Living"* chapter, but overall, red meat is nutrient-rich and high in quality protein and healthy fat. The current trend of replacing meat with processed alternatives deprives the body of necessary nutrients and replaces healthy fats with empty carbohydrates.

The fact is human beings evolved by, and came to thrive upon, consuming the muscles and organs of a variety of animals, including large ruminants like cattle. Red meat is an excellent source of:

- **Vitamin B12**, which is vital to mental and physical health, especially in protecting the integrity of nerves and the cardiovascular system
- **Vitamin D**, and particularly a partially metabolized form called 25-hydroxycholecalciferol, which is much more easily assimilated than the forms of vitamin D one gets in supplements
- **Iron**, in a form called heme iron. This is more readily absorbed than the nonheme iron found in plant foods
- **Saturated fat**, the kind of fat your body needs. Saturated fat is structurally sound fat—and since the membranes of your cells are made of fat, it pays to make them out of this solid, rather than liquid, form of fatty acid.

And just last year, red meat was shown beneficial for fat loss as well:

A recent analysis of data from the United States National Health and Nutrition Examination Survey (NHANES) reported that adults who eat red meat tend to have a lower body mass index and a smaller waist, eat more vegetables, and are less likely to suffer from hypertension than those adults who do not eat red meat.

Unprocessed red meats are a terrific source of high-quality protein, promoting healthy growth in children and healthy weight in adults. A report from *The American Journal of Clinical Nutrition* shows that higher-protein diets markedly increase satiety, meaning that you don't need to eat as much to get and stay full. The Meat Science report also examines data from NHANES, concluding that "increasing protein from 15% to 25% of energy intake in an obese individual would be expected to be associated with a decrease in energy intake of:

438 calories/day if protein is substituted for carbohydrates

620 calories/day if protein is substituted for fat."[30]

Eat more protein and fats from healthy animals and you will eat fewer carbs—the very things leading to weight gain.

## STEPS TO FREEDOM

1. Start your day with two cups of green tea to bump up your antioxidants and stimulate your metabolism.
2. Eat half of a fresh grapefruit before a meal.
3. Grind up some green veggies in water and drink a shot before a meal.
4. Don't shy away from spicy foods and peppers—the capsaicin will increase your fat-burning potential.
5. Make sure you're getting an adequate amount of vitamin D— if you don't spend roughly an hour a day outdoors between 10 a.m. and 3 p.m., include fish at least three times a week in your diet or consider taking a supplement.
6. Stock up on coconut oil—take it on its own, or use it as a replacement for other fats in your cooking to be sure you're getting a healthy dose each day.
7. Eat healthy, animal-based foods. Adding meat to your diet will help increase your feelings of satiety while providing you with healthy fats and other nutrients.

---

30 "Trends in carbohydrate, fat, and protein intakes and association with energy intake in nor-mal-weight, overweight, and obese individuals: 1971–2006." The American Journal of Clinical Nutrition. Web.

# NATURAL FOOD FLAVORS EXPOSED:

## Why Hidden Ingredients Impact Your Fat Loss and How to Avoid Them

I come from a long line of Oregon farmers and cattle ranchers, and I vividly recall how up until the 1960s, mixed-use family farms rotated cattle, grain, and vegetable crops with a nitrogen-fixing cover crop. This sustainable system kept soil fertile and delivered a healthy level of nutrients to the plants and animals.

I must emphasize "vividly recall" because your average modern-day food production Goliath bears little resemblance to the sort of farm we picture when we think of the word.

Studies show today's foods contain a mere fraction of the vitamins and minerals they did over 50 years ago. That's problem No 1.

Problem No. 2 is our convenience-worshiping culture, which has virtually eliminated home cooking in favor of canned, frozen, shrink-wrapped, or otherwise highly processed prepackaged foods.

Trouble is, these ready-made meals must taste good for people to come back for more, even though the processing usually strips any semblance of a pleasing flavor from the original ingredients. And when the crops themselves are virtually tasteless to start with because they are grown in nutrient-depleted soil, chances are slim the resulting product will taste better than drywall spackling paste.

Enter "natural flavors."

Look on any processed food's ingredient label and chances are you'll see that reassuring but intentionally vague term. The reality is these additives are anything but natural, and (indirectly, at the very least) they can ruin your fat-loss efforts.

If you want to do everything possible to ensure your fat-burning success, you must eliminate these additives from your diet. This guide will reveal:

- Exactly what they are . . .
- Where they're hidden . . .
- And how you can avoid them successfully.

The first thing that you should know is that if food declares itself to be "low-sugar," "low-sodium," or "fat-free," artificial flavors have almost certainly been added to replicate the taste of the real sugar, salt, or fat that's been removed.

But that's no problem, right? After all, the replacement is "natural flavoring," suggesting it's at least as healthy as the natural stuff that's been processed out. While the phrase might lead you to believe these are simple, healthy additions—an extra dose of garlic or cinnamon, for instance—the reality is actually quite disgusting.

According to the FDA's Code of Federal Regulations:

> The term *natural flavor* or *natural flavoring* means the essential oil, oleoresin, essence or extractive, protein hydrolysate, distillate, or any product of roasting, heating or enzymolysis, which contains the flavoring constituents derived from a spice, fruit or fruit juice, vegetable or vegetable juice, edible yeast, herb, bark, bud, root, leaf or similar plant material, meat, seafood, poultry, eggs, dairy products, or fermentation products thereof, whose significant function in food is flavoring rather than nutritional.

OK, got it? No? Don't worry, neither did I the first five or six times I tried to decipher it.

The take-home message is: Natural flavors are not always natural, and more often than not have little to do with the taste of the natural ingredient they're trying to emulate.

The FDA does not require manufacturers to list the ingredients in their "natural flavoring," so exactly what you're eating can be difficult to determine. For example, many "natural" raspberry flavors include castoreum, which is a yellow secretion beaver glands release along with urine to mark their territory. Not exactly what comes to mind when you think of raspberries, is it?

(Of course, while the FDA is loose as a goose in this realm, they're quite strict when it comes to outlawing the sale of milk in its natural, unpasteurized form. Nice guys, huh?)

What's more, these flavors can be quite addictive, leading you to crave and eat more than you normally would. Let's look at artificial sweeteners as an example.

Widely used in sports and energy drinks, along with sodas, sweeteners like aspartame have become a large part of the American diet.

Unfortunately, despite being labelled as "natural" flavoring, aspartame is essentially toxic. The secret lies in methanol, which makes up about 10% of aspartame. Methanol is converted to formaldehyde when it crosses the blood-brain barrier and can cause migraines, brain damage, vision problems, birth defects, and much more.

Aspartame is promoted as a healthy alternative to sugar and is used in diet sodas and sports drinks to promote weight loss. However, a study out of the University of Toronto, as well as many others, has shown that beverages with aspartame actually increase appetite.[31]

Why? Because taste and appetite work together in an elegant way. When you take a big swig of aspartame-sweetened soda, your metabolism immediately begins to anticipate a huge influx of calories. After all, for over a million years of evolution, the taste of sweetness has always been followed by a flood of carbohydrate, which the body handles by ramping up insulin production.

When you consume noncaloric sweetener, this ancient system is thrown completely out of whack. When a sweet taste is followed by zero calories, you begin to immediately crave calories in any form, from any source, to satisfy the intense craving.

Little wonder that no credible study has ever found that diet soda assists with weight loss.

Monosodium glutamate, usually called MSG, is a neurotoxin with known dangerous health effects and a profound impact on obesity, and is also an ingredient masked by the "natural flavor" title. Just another case of the food industry choosing profits over safety.

---

31 "Consuming aspartame with and without taste: differential effects on appetite and food intake of young adult males." Physiology & Behavior. Web.

This, however, only scratches the surface of so-called "natural" flavoring affecting your health and weight.

For decades, clever scientists have been studying the subtleties of food flavoring. They had to. As I pointed out before, whenever a processed food is created and stuffed into a bag or box and stabilized to spend months on a shelf, many of the assembled elements lose their natural flavor.

So (naturally) food companies scrambled to add this flavor back in, using concentrated extracts in specific dosages.

But why stop there?

As long as they were adding in flavoring agents, these food companies took the next logical (for them) step: manipulate the ratio of various flavoring agents to make it virtually impossible for you to stop eating.

With the right addictive flavor, minus the healthy fats or complex carbs that might actually satisfy you, these scientists cracked the code on getting you to crunch through an entire bag of puffs, curls, or chips without even realizing it!

An excellent expose on this natural flavoring fraud is detailed in an episode of *60 Minutes* called "The Flavorists," in which an all-too-agreeable Morley Safer ambles along with the professionals as they demonstrate, step by step, exactly what they do, and how.[32]

They are, in their own words, trying to make eating a "memorable" and "addictive" experience. It's their goal to make you want more. They design the flavors to be powerful but not linger too long, so that you keep going back for another taste.

So while the flavoring agents themselves don't make you fat, the carb-intensive foods to which they are added do. Without these flavorings, you wouldn't have any problem putting down a bag of chips unfinished. In fact, you'd never take more than one bite.

---

32 "The Flavorists: Tweaking Tastes and Creating Cravings." CBS News. Web.

## STEPS TO FREEDOM

So how to avoid these decidedly unnatural flavors?

It's not easy . . . but the results are worth it.

Start by looking at the ingredient label.

In the words of Morley Safer, "Most of the wrong stuff we eat comes in a bottle, a can, or a box—food that's been processed. Much of that food has been flavored. The flavoring industry is the enabler of the food-processing business, which depends upon it to create a craving for everything from soda pop to chicken soup."

Most ingredient labels disguise this deception by simply listing "natural flavors." Even seemingly healthy brands contain this mystery element.

So remember: There's no free lunch, flavored or otherwise. Convenient, prepackaged foods come with a price in the form of addictive additives. If you want real fat-loss results, you must stick to eating real foods.

In the past, this was all but impossible, considering most of the hearty, filling natural foods were banished to the government's "foods to minimize" list. Actually, they still are, but now you know better.

That's the big picture. But here are some more specific pro tips to make all this easy:

1. Eat foods that don't have labels at all, like produce and fresh organic meat.
2. If you must eat something labeled, avoid anything with more than seven ingredients, words you don't recognize, or the term "natural flavors."
3. Avoid anything labeled "diet," "low-fat" or "low-sugar," since the substitutes for those sugars and fats are often worse than what they replace.

# LIQUID POISON EXPOSED:
## Avoid This Insidious Fat-Gainer

If you're trying to lose weight, there's one thing in your diet that you should eliminate, without question.

In fact, this beverage is so dangerous that I refer to it as "liquid poison."

The problem is this particular poison seems to be an integral part of our national identity. It's as big a part of Americana as apple pie and fireworks on the Fourth of July. The biggest brands dominate our commercials and billboards, selling their poison as the key to happiness and refreshment.

I'm talking about soda.

In 2001, Americans gulped down 135% more of this poison than in 1977, an increase that's in near-perfect lock step with our obesity epidemic. The good news is a study looking at our consumption from 1999–2010 showed a slight trend down.[33] The bad news is it didn't also count fruit juices, which can spike blood sugar as much as soda. And it didn't count "energy drinks," which are nothing more than highly caffeinated soda.

So overall, sweet, unhealthy drinks remain on the rise.

But let's keep the focus on classic sweetened soda, which is still consumed at the horrifying rate of *44 gallons* per American annually.

---

33 "Trends in sugar-sweetened beverage consumption among youth and adults in the United States: 1999–2010." The American Journal of Clinical Nutrition. Web.

A little-known study showed this liquid poison can start jacking up your weight in just three weeks.[34] Another showed adding soda into your diet can cause a three-pound weight gain in 10 weeks.[35] These numbers might not seem significant, until you consider these effects are due to soda alone, *without any other diet changes*.

In other words, it's strong enough to wreak havoc all on its own.

Another study showed it causes more weight gain than stuffing your face with the same number of calories from jelly beans . . . *jelly beans!*[36]

Think of it this way:

Every time you drink soda, you might as well be programming your DNA to transform your body into a fat-storing machine.

Don't be dramatic, you might be thinking. I drink only diet soda—there are no sugar and no calories in a diet soda!

You're right about that. But what they use to replace the sugar and calories is even worse.

*Prevention* cites a University of Minnesota study of 10,000 adults which found that "even just one diet soda a day was linked to a 34% higher risk of metabolic syndrome, a group of symptoms including belly fat and high cholesterol that put you at risk for heart disease." Diet soda also has been linked to kidney disease and reproductive issues.

Overall, it appears that the artificial sweeteners in soda are at least as bad for you as actual sugar.

This secret might seem a little basic or obvious to some folks. But I'm compelled to include this guide in **Freedom From Fat** because Americans are *still* consuming an insane volume of soda.

Notice something wrong with the numbers in the chart on the next page? I do . . .

**They're not ZERO!**

When I'm feeling unusually masochistic, I stroll down the soda aisle in a supermarket, just to get a feel for the sugar-soaked metabolic nightmares disguised as innocent groceries.

---

34 "Effect of drinking soda sweetened with aspartame or high fructose corn syrup on food intake and body weight." The American Journal of Clinical Nutrition. Web.

35 "Sucrose compared with artificial sweeteners: different effects on ad libitum food intake and body weight after 10 wk of supplementation in overweight subjects." The American Journal of Clinical Nutrition. Web.

36 "Liquid versus solid carbohydrate: effects on food intake and body weight." Obesity. Web.

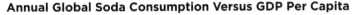

### Annual Global Soda Consumption Versus GDP Per Capita

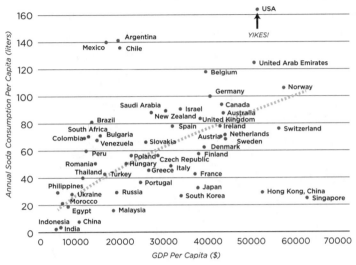

Source: Credit Suisse Research Institute

They shouldn't even exist. Because the correct amount of soda every man, woman and child on this planet should drink for health is:

0

Zilch.

Nada.

As in . . . never again!

## STEPS TO FREEDOM

Perform an exorcism on your kitchen. Pour all soda down the drain as if you were an addict determined to go straight (which may be close to the truth). Don't feel any guilt for wasting it, because it has no food value whatsoever.

If soda's currently in your diet, eliminating this single item will make it far easier to drop fat from your body.

Replace it with water or unsweetened green or black tea for hydration. You can also have a cup of coffee or two daily—it's rich in antioxidants and may also accelerate your metabolism, making fat burning a little easier. You can put some half and half in it, but skip the sweeteners!

That's it. No juice. No energy drinks. No sweet liquids of any kind.

Don't make the mistake of replacing one sugar bomb for another.

You might feel symptoms of withdrawal . . . which should give you a hint of how horrible this stuff is for your health. I assure you, those pains will pass, and you'll feel (and look!) better for it.

# THE FOOD TIMING TRICK TO ACCELERATE FAT LOSS

I'm sure you've heard the supposedly sage advice "Eat five or six small meals per day" for health and weight loss. As a young man in the 1970s, I never heard anyone suggest this, but these days, it's close to nutritional dogma. An online search of the phrase "eat many small meals" returns over 275,000 results!

Maybe you've even passed this advice along yourself.

If so, consider yourself forgiven. Because "gems" like these are buried so deep in our psyches that we seldom think to question—much less reject—their basic premises.

But in this case, you might want to explore whether this whole "many small meals" thing is the real deal . . . or just common senselessness.

When people are told to "eat many small meals," what they hear is "eat all the time," an activity at which most Americans excel.

It's no coincidence that obesity rates started ratcheting skyward in the 1980s, more or less in tandem with this widespread endorsement of more frequent meals. (The other major culprit was the government's nonsensical "low-fat, high-carb" dietary recommendation, which also leads to excessive hunger and chronic overeating).

In my overseas travels, I rarely see people chowing down in their cars or in line for a movie or otherwise outside the traditional time and space boundaries of a meal. In the U.S., it seems that everyone continually eats everywhere.

Bad news: The theory of eating five or six meals per day for health and weight loss . . . is pure moonshine.

And the good news (I like to end on a high note): A slight tweak to this theory could actually *be one of the best-kept secrets for fat burning*. More on that in a moment. First let's demolish the myth of noshing on nuggets of food throughout the day:

One study out of the Netherlands' Maastricht University Medical Center evaluated the differences in a low-frequency diet of three meals per day versus a high-frequency diet of 14 small meals per day.[37]

Although the low-frequency diet did result in more drastic fluctuations in insulin levels (higher highs and lower lows), there was no difference in energy expenditure between the diets. This means that there was no weight-loss benefit to eating smaller, more frequent meals.

The researchers believe that this might be because "the insulin levels did not increase high enough to inhibit fat oxidation in the [high-frequency diet]." In other words, since their insulin and glucose were continuously at the same level, there was no signal to switch on the body's fat-burning machinery.

Furthermore, they found that the low-frequency diet led to lower blood sugar levels, which led the researchers to suggest that "this can lead to a better body weight control on the long term."

A low-frequency diet of three meals per day led to greater feelings of satiety (in other words, fullness), meaning that the subjects were not hungry throughout the day and practiced better appetite control. These same results have been found in trials of young, healthy males as well as obese males when eating a high-protein diet.

And it gets worse for the whole "many meals" thing: A small study measured the blood glucose levels of subjects eating three high-carb meals in a day, six high-carb meals, or six high-protein meals.[38] Glucose remained elevated longer throughout the day for those eating six high-carb meals. Chronically high blood glucose could lead to insulin resistance, often a preliminary step toward Type 2 diabetes. If you get that, a few extra

---

37 "Effects of Meal Frequency on Metabolic Profiles and Substrate Partitioning in Lean Healthy Males." PLOS One. Web.

38 "Effect of Meal Frequency on Glucose and Insulin." Elsevier. Web.

pounds around your belly will be the least of your worries.

Chronically high glucose levels will also help keep you addicted to Big Food's products, so don't expect a peep from these industrial carb pushers about decreasing how frequently you eat.

## SO WHAT'S THE ANSWER?

Certainly not starvation.

The Department of Medicine at the University of Rochester School of Medicine and Dentistry looked at the differences between short and prolonged fasting.[39] They found that resting metabolic rates fell an average of 8% after three days of fasting, including the percent of carbohydrates and protein being metabolized.

But . . . this was after three days.

A long-term fast can have negative effects on your metabolism. Studies have shown that it's fat-burning potential spikes in the early stages of fasting and then evens out. Prolonging your starvation won't continue to spike your metabolic rate.

Short-term fasting, on the other hand, optimizes these increases, resting energy expenditure.

One easy strategy is called "alternate-day modified fasting." That simply means you limit your caloric intake every other day of the week. Then on the days you're not fasting, eat as much as you please.

This method is also more effective than regular dieting. One study from the Shahid Beheshti University of Medical Sciences in Tehran, Iran studied 74 people, comparing a "calorie shifting diet" (intermediate fasting) with a classic calorie-restrictive diet.[40] They found that the calorie shifting diet had greater improvement, resulting in a decrease in hunger and an increase in satisfaction after meals after the subjects dieted for four weeks.

The results of intermittent, or alternate-day fasting, can be incredible.

You do need to keep in mind what you're eating or how often. Stick to a high-fat, moderate protein, low-carb diet for the best results.

---

39 "Leucine, glucose, and energy metabolism after 3 days of fasting in healthy human subjects." The American Journal of Clinical Nutrition. Web.

40 "Calorie shifting diet versus calorie restriction diet: a comparative clinical trial study." International Journal of Preventative Medicine.

Otherwise, the sugars in the carbohydrates you consume will affect your insulin levels, negating the benefits of the fast.

## OK, SO IT'S GOOD FOR FAT LOSS . . . BUT WHAT ABOUT HEALTH?

Many people who read about intermittent fasting bring up an important question:

"Even if I can drop fat rapidly, isn't it bad for my health to go without food for so many hours per day?"

If you're concerned about that, then here's a word that I humbly suggest you add to your healthy-living vocabulary.

It's *autophagy*, pronounced aw-TAW-fug-ee.

Coined by Belgian biochemist and Nobel Prize winner Christian de Duve in 1963, it combines the Greek *auto-*, signifying "self-," and *phagein*, which means "to eat."

Understanding what it is, and how to optimize it, is absolutely vital.

Autophagy happens continually within all multicelled creatures. That includes you and me, a couple of 37 trillion cell arrangements popularly known as human beings.

As we create new cells by the millions hourly, we must also carry out autophagy—disposal of the dying and dead cells via "self-eating."

The efficiency of your autophagous machinery is vastly important to your health.

During this process, lysosomes—tiny sphere-shaped structures inside each cell—spew out about 40 kinds of enzymes to break apart decaying proteins and other big molecules into smaller, simpler ones that can be used to build new cells.

Lysosomes also help to destroy disease-causing bacteria and viruses.

As with any bodily process, autophagy can be vigorous, average, or seriously screwed up. This matters. The efficiency of your autophagous machinery is vastly important to your health.

Robust autophagy leads to long life. Indeed, while you'll hear millions of claims that this diet or that behavior can extend life, optimal autophagy is one of the few scientifically confirmed processes that can do this.

In animal studies, life spans have been extended up to 65%.

Ramped-up autophagy has also been shown in studies to lower risk of cancer, insulin resistance, infection, heart disease, neurodegenerative diseases (such as Parkinson's and Alzheimer's), and inflammation in general.

A 2006 study by Johnson, Laub, and John states:

> Since May 2003, we have experimented with alternate-day calorie restriction, one day consuming 20–50% of estimated daily caloric requirement and the next day ad lib [the technical term for "unrestricted"] eating, and have observed health benefits starting in as little as two weeks, in insulin resistance; asthma; seasonal allergies; infectious diseases of viral, bacterial, and fungal origin (viral URI, recurrent bacterial tonsillitis, chronic sinusitis, periodontal disease); autoimmune disorder (rheumatoid arthritis); osteoarthritis; symptoms due to CNS inflammatory lesions (Tourette's, Meniere's); cardiac arrhythmias (PVCs, atrial fibrillation); [and] menopause-related hot flashes.[41]

So now you know, not only is intermittent fasting great for fat loss, it can also help you build robust health.

## STEPS TO FREEDOM

**1. Get hungry now and then.** "One well-recognized way of inducing autophagy is by food restriction, which upregulates autophagy in many organs," concludes a 2010 study from the Scripps Research Institute in La Jolla, California.

In other words, practice intermittent fasting! Skip one meal a day, or one day of solid food per week. Perhaps the simplest tactic is to eat only within a six-hour "window" from noon to 6 p.m. Do what works in your life. "Hungrying up" on a regular basis matters more than the precise form and timing.

Of the three steps I'm going to present here, this first step is the most effective. Yet mainstream health advice often advises just the opposite.

---

41 "The effect on health of alternate day calorie restriction: Eating less and more than needed on alternate days prolongs life." Medical Hypotheses. Web.

Now, I realize that disciplined eating is not easy. I like to chow down as much as, and perhaps more than, the next guy. But I've found it helps me to power through bouts of hunger to imagine leagues of industrious lysosomes busily power-washing accumulated junk out of my tissues.

Make hunger your friend. Regularly embracing even mild hunger can ultimately bring not only physical health but also mental focus and improved mood . . . and, of course, more effective fat loss. It's worth the effort.

**2. Eat a high-fat, moderate-protein, low-carbohydrate diet.** As I've written previously, carbohydrates will spike your glucose levels and lead to problems like chronic inflammation and insulin resistance . . . yes, even the darling so-called "heart-healthy whole grains" we've been duped into making the foundation of our diets.

Avoid them at all costs. Follow a diet high in healthy fats for the best results.

Most importantly, make sure to adjust your diet to contain more healthy fats *before* you engage in any kind of intermittent fasting. If you try to skip meals first, you run the risk of carb addiction getting the better of you, which will make for an unpleasant experience. For this food timing trick to work, you need a satisfied appetite, and eating fat creates one.

**3. Exercise.** We all know exercise can make us healthy, but why? Its ability to boost autophagy appears to be the major reason. During exercise, virtually every kind of tissue experiences a boost in lysosome activity.

Combine exercise, especially the kind described in **Lightning-Fast Fat Loss**, with this food timing trick and you just might experience the most rapid fat loss of your life.

# LIGHTNING-FAST FAT LOSS:
## Turbocharge Your Fat-Burning 900% With This Cutting-Edge Fitness Technique

### WHY WORK OUT FOR HOURS WHEN MINUTES WILL DO?

Almost 20 years ago, while most fitness-minded Americans were dutifully grinding out hours of mind-numbing aerobic exercise, a researcher named Dr. Izumi Tabata quietly published some intriguing experimental results based on an unusual training regimen of the Japanese speed skating team.[42]

The head coach wanted to see, in real numbers, just how effective his training was. The results were so startling, they created a sensation in the word of fitness research. "Although Coach Irisawa pioneered the idea, somehow it became named after me," Dr. Tabata wryly observed.

Thus, the Tabata Protocol was born.

Dr. Tabata discovered that working out for mere minutes, but at a more intense level, could be more beneficial than spending hours at the gym.

According to a study published in *The Journal of Physiology*, Dr. Tabata was on to something: 16 healthy young men were split into two groups.[43] The first group performed four–six 30-second bursts of exercise (with four minutes of recovery between their efforts). The second slogged it out for 90–120 minutes of steady, moderate exertion on an exercise bike gizmo.

---

42 "Effects of moderate-intensity endurance and high-intensity intermittent training on anaerobic capacity and VO2max." Medicine and Science in Sports and Exercise. Web.

43 "Short-term sprint interval versus traditional endurance training: similar initial adaptations in human skeletal muscle and exercise performance." The Journal of Physiology. Web.

At the end of two weeks, the high-intensity group had exercised for about 2½ hours total, including the recovery periods. The slow-and-steady group had logged over 10 hours.

When muscle biopsies were performed to measure the results of the training, the conclusion was nothing short of revolutionary. The stationary bikers were wasting their time (or, more accurately, about 75% of it). Why? Because the skeletal muscle adaptations and exercise performance between the groups were virtually identical.

It sounds impossible, but all of this makes good sense from an evolutionary perspective. High-intensity training tells your body that survival in this environment requires extraordinary speed and strength. (Your body doesn't believe you are crazy enough to work this hard otherwise.) It responds by marshaling metabolically "expensive" muscle-building and fat-burning mechanisms to make you a lean, mean survival machine.

Conversely, slow jogs or swims lack urgency. Loathe to waste energy on dramatic changes, your body assumes that partial adaption will do. Result: Months of workouts slide by and progress remains nearly undetectable.

The take-home point for you is don't bother horsewhipping yourself on a bike, treadmill, or running path for hours on end. Instead of wasting months training for a marathon, train for just a few minutes and bank the rest of that time doing . . . well, whatever you'd like!

There's even more compelling research on the merits of workouts that are short in duration but high in intensity. Incredibly, even a three-minute workout can have the same benefit as one lasting 90 minutes–two hours.

The science also shows this form of training is, bar none, the best for burning fat.

A University of Virginia study tested volunteers in three groups: One sat on its collective duff the entire time.[44] The second performed long, slow aerobic exercise. And the third performed more intense exercise with a shorter duration.

---

44 "Effect of exercise training intensity on abdominal visceral fat and body composition." National Institute of Health. Web.

One (and only one) group managed to burn away significant amounts of belly fat. It wasn't the couch potatoes, and it wasn't those doing typical aerobics. Once again, the shorter, more intense workouts reigned supreme.

Another interesting result: The metabolic rate of the low-intensity exercisers actually went down during the study. The more intense exercisers achieved faster metabolisms.

But you didn't just fall off the radicchio truck. You're looking for the catch.

Indeed, there is one.

As one researcher put it, you must commit to spending most of that brief high-exertion interval at an "8 or above" on a 1–10 intensity scale.

In other words—and excuse the vernacular—you need to seriously bust ass.

This sort of exercise is known as high-intensity interval training, or HIIT. It has long been known to serious athletes but is now finally entering the mainstream.

The same research group that did the study above found in another that HIIT burned fat more efficiently than did typical aerobics. They tracked two groups. One performed 20 weeks of conventional aerobics, and the other did 15 weeks of HIIT.

The first group burned more calories per workout session, *but the second group incinerated an astounding 900% more fat.*

So why isn't this form of fitness more popular?

Other than the requisite ass-busting (this really does need to be emphasized), many people are turned off because they've been lulled into chasing something called the "fat-burning zone" when they exercise.

Perhaps you've seen this seductive term on a poster near the treadmills at the gym. The poster may also feature a fancy-colored graph marking off certain percentages of maximum heart rate.

The idea is simple (and, as you'll soon discover, rather misleading): Keep your heart rate, and intensity, within 55–65% of maximum and you'll burn fat at maximum efficiency during your workout.

Sounds fantastic! But there are two major flaws:

1. While exercising at a lower, more comfortable intensity for a longer duration will burn a greater *percentage* of fat, the total amount is still miniscule. Higher-intensity workouts burn more total calories, including after you're finished. This is in contrast to your typical boring, endless cardio, which only seems to increase your appetite after you're done. This means, all things being equal, more fat will disappear from your body.

2. Higher-intensity workouts boost the release of human growth hormone (HGH), which acts like a youth serum in your body, firming muscles, tightening skin, increasing energy, improving sleep . . . and carving away fat. Low-intensity exercise causes little or no release of HGH.

This second point was confirmed by Dr. Christopher Scott at the University of Southern Maine. He examined the differences between steady cycling and 15-minute sprints and found the sprinters burned 95% of their calories *after the exercise was over.*[45]

Bottom line: Slashing the time and pumping up the intensity can give you dramatically better exercise results.

## SO IS HIIT FOR YOU?

That depends. While it delivers faster benefits, it requires a certain mental toughness that some people just can't muster.

If you're in that group, keep taking long walks, leisurely bike rides, and placid swims. These are far better than doing nothing. For those who have the time, these can build a strong conditioning foundation.

Another important caveat—HIIT can hurt you. Anyone with any reason to suspect susceptibility to heart attack should remain well below the "8 on a scale of 1–10" territory.

But for me personally, HIIT has been a revelation. I was a serious runner for many years, dutifully logging up to 50 miles a week, yet the spare tire hung on stubbornly.

---

45 "Afterburn Effect: Burn 500+ Calories from 10 Minutes of Exercise?" Built Lean. Web.

So for the last five years or so, I've been doing HIIT and mixing up the activity. When running, I alternate between block-long sprints and rests. When biking, it's one minute flat-out and then 15 seconds easy, for a quick four miles to my office.

But swimming according to an HIIT regime has been the most satisfying of all. Where I once cranked out a steady, moderate-paced, mind-numbing half mile, these days I do a series of six laps of our small pool at maximum speed and then 30 seconds of rest.

The last half of the sixth lap is utterly brutal, but I keep in mind that it will be over soon! And not only do I stop after six laps, but I actually exit the pool, soak up the sun for 30 seconds, and then hop in and go again.

A workout consisting of six six-lap sessions and five quick rests takes no more than 20 minutes and leaves me pleasantly exhausted. I'm glad to report the spare tire is long gone.

You need not do HIIT exclusively. Long walks and placid swims are still part of my life and a nice counterpoint to HIIT's intensity.

But try it at least a couple of times a week. Trim and toned, you and I can then return to our sedentary jobs guilt-free (though I have a stand-up desk, so I am not a total slug at work—standing burns twice as many calories as sitting).

## STEPS TO FREEDOM

1. Resolve to make HIIT a part of your life, even if it seems strange and you're nervous about doing so. It might help your motivation to review all the fat-burning and health benefits:
   - You can finish the workout almost 10 times faster than you can with regular cardio but get better fat-burning results
   - It increases your fat burning for the rest of the day
   - It increases your youth-associated hormones like HGH
   - It releases endorphins, which give you a "feel good" sensation to enjoy after your workout is over
   - It makes any of your other workouts more efficient for burning fat
   - It simultaneously molds muscle and increases heart health.

2. Break into HIIT gently if you're not experienced. It's counterintuitive, but tougher forms of HIIT like running uphill or carrying extra weights can be safer, because your speed will go down.

3. Learn to appreciate the challenge. Remember, the benefits of HIIT come *specifically* from how tough it is. So there's no "getting around" the hard workout aspect of it. You're just going to have to learn to love it, which will get surprisingly easy when you see the results in the mirror and relish how fantastic you feel after you're done.

Plus, remember: These workouts are short, and you must have at least a two-day break between them. With HIIT, you can put to rest the idea of slogging it out on the treadmill or pounding the pavement every day. Instead, you'll be burning fat 900% more efficiently. Use the free time to enjoy your new body!

# CHEAT SHEET

I've given you plenty of good news in this report. Many of the foods that you've been avoiding (and missing) are actually beneficial for your health. Saturated fats can be put back on your menu, allowing you to indulge.

However, I do realize that by exposing these health secrets, I've taken a few things away from you. Grains, carbohydrates, white flour, and sugars have come to permeate our diets for a reason: They're delicious!

I do stand by the fact that they should be avoided. One famous science journalist who helped to change the conversation about saturated fats is Gary Taubes. In his book *Good Calories, Bad Calories*, Taubes "argued that refined carbohydrates and sugars in our diet are what cause obesity, diabetes, and related diseases, and not the dietary fat or the 'excess calories' that are thought to come from eating more than we should."

He, along with many other nutritionists and scientists who are starting to see the light, believes that insulin contributes largely to obesity. And insulin spikes when you eat carbohydrates.

But what if you like foods like pancakes, mashed potatoes, and pizza? It might not be enough for us to give you steak and take away all of these delicious treats.

I will show you how you can STILL enjoy those foods without risking your health. As I mentioned, the steak and wine diet is about doing what you enjoy . . . it's not a painful, lose-20-pounds-fast solution. It's about loving life and being good to your body.

I know it's not easy to significantly lower your carb consumption, even if you do get to have steak and butter in their place. To try to make that a little easier for you, I have assembled some well-tested recipes for you below.

These are all great for you, and taste delicious as well.

## PANCAKES

Pancakes have long been frowned upon as an unhealthy breakfast choice. Unfortunately, with their high carb content, I'd have to agree in saying that you should steer clear of traditional pancakes for breakfast. However, by substituting the white flour with healthy alternatives, you avoid an unnecessary insulin spike early in the morning.

### Almond Flour Pancakes—from PrimalPalate.com

**Ingredients:**

1¾ cup blanched almond flour
2 pastured eggs, whisked
½ tsp salt
1 tsp pure vanilla extract
½ tsp ground cinnamon
¼ tsp ground nutmeg
1 cup water
1 tbsp salted butter, for frying

**Directions:**

1. In a small mixing bowl, whisk two eggs.

2. Pour almond flour, salt, cinnamon, and nutmeg into a medium-sized mixing bowl.

3. Add vanilla extract and eggs to the bowl.

4. Mix with a wooden spoon to combine.

5. Add water, and continue to stir.

6. Heat 1 tablespoon of grass-fed butter or coconut oil in a large nonstick skillet.

7. Using 1/8 cup, scoop batter into the frying pan, leaving enough space in between pancakes to flip.

8. Cook 2 minutes on the first side, flip, and cook for a remaining 1–2 minutes. Add additional cooking fat as needed. (It helps to flip pancakes back and forth a bit to ensure they are cooked through.)

9. Top with your choice of grass-fed butter or coconut oil, and a sprinkle of cinnamon, and serve.

## Banana Pancakes

**Ingredients:**

1 egg
2 tbsps almond butter
2 ripe bananas
Shredded coconut
Coconut oil
Ground cinnamon
Honey (if desired)

**Directions:**

1. Mash the two bananas with a fork. Get the texture to your preference — it's OK to leave it a little lumpy, if you don't mind it.

2. Crack the egg into the banana mixture, mixing it in.

3. Add almond butter, shredded coconut, and a sprinkle of cinnamon. The coconut will just help hold the batter together— you can play around with how much you would like to add.

4. Heat either coconut oil or butter in a frying pan.

5. Scoop in the batter, keeping on a low heat. The pancakes will be ready to flip once bubbles rise to the top. Generally, it takes about 2–3 minutes on each side.

6. Drizzle honey over the pancakes and enjoy!

**Added benefit:** Cinnamon is proven to be great for helping to keep your blood sugar at a more consistent level. In this case, it will be great to balance the sugar from the bananas.

## SANDWICH BREAD—from guiltykitchen.com

One of the biggest struggles I've personally had with this diet is the absence of bread. An English muffin for breakfast and a sandwich for lunch are easy, accessible meals that I used to believe were healthy.

Luckily, if you can't give that up, there are plenty of "breadless breads" out there. Below is one recipe I've grown to love.

**Ingredients:**

3/4 cup soaked almond butter, smooth *(store-bought works fine too)*
6 pastured eggs
2 tbsp honey
1/4 cup coconut oil, melted
1/2 tsp apple cider vinegar
1/4 cup ground golden flax
3 tbsp coconut flour
1 tsp baking soda
1/2 tsp sea salt

**Directions:**

1. Preheat oven to 350 degrees F. Line an 8x4-inch loaf pan with parchment, grease well with coconut oil.

2. In a large bowl, blend the almond butter, eggs, honey, coconut oil, and apple cider vinegar with an immersion blender.

3. In a separate bowl, combine the flax, coconut flour, baking soda, and sea salt. Mix the dry into the wet, pour into the greased and lined loaf pan, and bake for 35–40 minutes.

4. Remove from oven and allow to cool in pan 10 minutes. Remove from pan by pulling up on the parchment. Set on wire rack to cool completely.

5. Store in an airtight container at room temperature for 3–4 days, in the fridge for 7–10 days, or in the freezer for a month or so.

## PIZZA

Perhaps the ultimate "sin food," any dietician will be quick to tell you to avoid this delicious, cheesy, greasy pie. However, you now know that the real problem with pizza is the flour-intensive crust. However, there are ways to turn pizza into something that can be enjoyed not only for the taste, but also for the health benefits.

Don't be afraid when I introduce these two words: cauliflower crust.

Despite what you may think, cauliflower crust holds together nicely to form a slice that you can pick up and enjoy just like you would one from your local pizza shop.

And you can still include all of the toppings you love: cheese, bacon, veggies, you name it.

I'm going to give you a recipe for cauliflower crust that I think you'll really enjoy. This can sometimes take a few tries before you get it just right, so don't be discouraged! It's super simple once you get the hang of it.

**Ingredients:**

2 cups cauliflower
2 cups shaved mozzarella cheese
2 eggs

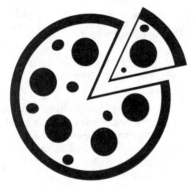

This is just one option for delicious, healthy pizza. For more great recipes, check out:

PaleoGrubs.com/pizza-recipes

**Directions:**

1. Preheat oven to 450 degrees F.

2. Grate the cauliflower or grind in a food processor.

3. Mix eggs, cauliflower, and mozzarella in a bowl. As you do, remove any larger chunks of cauliflower—they won't blend well.

4. Line a pizza pan with parchment paper—this helps prevent it from sticking. Don't oil the pan—cheese does that. Put "dough" mixture on the pan and evenly press it into a thin, round crust. Be sure to make it pretty thin.

5. Put in the oven for 15 minutes.

6. Then put toppings on—veggies, meat, sauces, as long as there's no sugar or high-fructose corn syrup. (We encourage a bacon and meat lover's pizza, personally.)

# CHEESY GARLIC BREAD—from cutthewheat.com

I don't know about you, but I am a sucker for garlic bread. Warm, cheesy, doughy foods have always been a weakness of mine, and this is no exception. Luckily, it's possible to make this treat without the bread!

**Ingredients (for bread base):**

1¼ cups almond flour
1 tbsp coconut flour
3 egg whites, beaten until fluffy
2 tbsp olive oil or avocado oil
1/4 cup warm water
1 tsp live yeast granules
1 tsp coconut sugar (or honey or molasses—will be eaten by yeast)
1/2 cup shredded mozzarella cheese
1/4 tsp salt
2 tsp baking powder
1/4 tsp garlic powder

**Ingredients (for topping):**

1 cup shredded mozzarella cheese
2 Tbsp butter, melted
1/4 tsp garlic powder
1/4 tsp salt
1/2 tsp Italian seasoning

**Directions:**

1. Preheat oven to 400 degrees F.

2. In a large bowl, combine almond and coconut flour, salt, baking powder, garlic powder, and xanthan gum. Stir well.

3. In a small cup or bowl, combine warm water and sugar and stir until dissolved, and then add yeast. Set aside for a few moments.

4. To the flour mixture, add olive oil and yeast-water mixture and stir well with a rubber spatula. Add in beaten eggs and continue to mix.

5. Add in the 1/2 cup mozzarella shreds and mix gently with your spatula until a nice dough is formed and cheese is mixed well throughout.

6. Grease a 9x9-inch square cake pan or large cookie sheet. Put batter into cake pan or cookie sheet. If you're free-forming on a cookie sheet, loosely form the dough into a rectangle or square.

7. Bake for approximately 15–17 minutes or until the sides of the crust turn golden brown. Remove and top.

8. In a small bowl, combine butter, garlic powder, and salt. Mix well and then brush over the top of the garlic bread base. Be sure to get the butter over every inch!

9. Top the bread with shredded mozzarella cheese, and then sprinkle that with Italian seasoning.

10. Bake for about 10 minutes or until cheese is melted. For final 3 minutes, turn broiler on to brown the cheese.

11. Remove from oven and let bread stand for 5–10 minutes before serving (if you can wait that long).

# PASTA

One of the most difficult parts of eating this way is the lack of pasta in my diet. Pasta is quick and easy to make, and can be prepared in so many ways that it keeps things interesting.

Luckily, you can still have the taste of the meals you love without the harmful carbohydrates. Below are two of my favorite recipes to help get around the pasta problem.

## Eggplant Lasagna

Lasagna, full of its rich, cheesy flavors, is one of my favorites. By substituting the noodle layers for eggplant, you can still have this delicious meal without the guilt.

**Ingredients:**

(Makes 8 servings)
2 large eggplants
Olive oil
Salt and ground black pepper—to taste
1 pound ground beef
48 ounces chunky tomato sauce
2 cups shredded mozzarella cheese
1 cup ricotta cheese

**Directions:**

1. Preheat oven to 375 degrees F. Oil two baking sheets.
2. Slice both eggplants into rounds, about ¼ inch thick.
3. Bake eggplant slices in the preheated oven for 20–25 minutes. Flip eggplant and bake an additional 20–25 minutes, until soft and golden brown.
4. Remove eggplant from the oven and increase temperature to 400 degrees F.
5. Heat butter in a skillet over medium-high heat and add ground beef. Season beef with salt and ground black pepper.
6. Cook and stir until beef is crumbly, evenly browned, and no longer pink, about 10 minutes. Drain excess grease.
7. Stir tomato sauce into ground beef; bring to a simmer and set sauce aside.
8. Lightly grease a 9x13-inch baking dish with coconut oil or butter
9. Place 1/3 of the eggplant slices on bottom of the dish.
10. Pour 1/3 of tomato sauce with ground beef on top of eggplant layer.
11. Sprinkle 1/3 of mozzarella cheese on top of sauce layer.
12. Spread ricotta cheese on top of mozzarella and sauce.
13. Repeat 2 more times, finishing with a layer of mozzarella cheese.
14. Bake uncovered in the preheated oven until cheese is melted and sauce is bubbling, 10–15 minutes.
15. Remove from oven and allow to cool for 5 minutes.

## Spaghetti Squash

Spaghetti squash is easy to prepare and can act as a substitute for pretty much any pasta dish you love. It comes out like an angel hair pasta—thin and delicate. It can be topped with anything you like: spaghetti and meatballs, pesto, carbonara, Alfredo—you name it!

Below are instructions on how to prepare the squash. From there, you can create any number of meals!

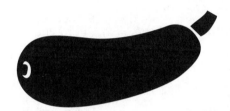

### Directions:
1. Preheat oven to 375 degrees F.
2. Cut the squash in half, lengthwise. It can be tough, so be sure to use a chef's knife.
3. Use a spoon to scoop out any seeds or excess, stringy flesh from the center. It will look a bit like a pumpkin once it's opened—it should be clear what to remove. Once you're done, it should be smooth.
4. Brush the inside of each half with butter and sprinkle with coarse salt and freshly ground black pepper.
5. Place cut sides down on a rimmed baking sheet, or in a roasting pan, and put into the oven.
6. Bake for about 40 minutes, or until you can easily pierce the squash with a fork.

## COOKIES

I hope you didn't think that I had forgotten about dessert.

You might be surprised to find that there are plenty of delicious dessert recipes out there that won't load you up with unnecessary carbs and sugars.

Below is one such recipe that I really think you'll enjoy, from 17Recipes.com.

**Ingredients:**

1/2 cup raisins
2½ cups hazelnut or almond flour
1 tsp baking soda
1/8 tsp salt
2 Tbsps coconut oil
1 egg
1 tsp vanilla extract
1/4 cup unsweetened coconut flakes
1/2 cup chocolate chips (make sure that you are using dark chocolate, with a high percentage of cacao content)

**Directions:**

1. Preheat oven to 350 degrees F.
2. Put raisins and flour in food processor, and blend until the raisins are finely chopped.
3. Add baking soda and salt and blend for a few pulses.
4. Add oil, egg, vanilla extract. Pulse until blended. Do not overblend, or the dough will get too greasy.
5. Mix chocolate chips and coconut flakes in by hand.
6. Place dough on cookie sheet— each ball of dough should be about the size of a walnut.
7. Bake for 8–10 minutes, until golden brown.

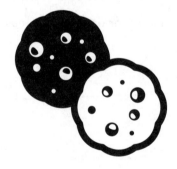

# NOTES